Energize Your Life

Navigating Wellness and Beating Fatigue

SEBASTIAN FERGUSON

Introduction

Fatigue had made an unpleasant appearance in the center of Selene's hectic existence, acting as an unwanted guest who stayed too long. As tiredness encircled her aspirations, desires, and even her happy moments, each day seemed to be a struggle. A guiding light, a ray of hope, however, may be found inside these pages that will enable Selene to not only face her exhaustion head-on but also to triumph over it, leaving her with newfound vigor and purpose.

The tale of Selene is not unusual. Fatigue can be a terrible foe in a world that asks so much of us—a world where we're expected to perform in our employment, nurture our relationships, and grow our passions. The story of Selene, however, changes today. Selene is about to go on a transforming journey with the help of the ideas, tactics, and useful advice presented in "Energize Your Life."

This book is more than a simple collection of words; it's a complete toolkit designed to relate to Selene's struggles and experiences. Each chapter provides a road map to restore her vitality, from identifying the root reasons of her exhaustion to making lifestyle adjustments that support her goals. Selene will learn how to get the most out of her sleep, take care of her health, and develop a mindset that gives her the strength to face challenges.

But Selene's transformation doesn't end with knowledge; real change is sparked by putting these ideas into practice. I urge Selene to interact with the exercises, think about her personal experiences, and picture the life she wants to live when the grip of exhaustion has been released. The challenge to take control of her own wellbeing and guide it toward a better, more energizing future is part of the call to action, which is more than just an invitation.

Selene and the knowledge contained in these pages will travel together on the path of conquering weariness. It's a journey that calls for dedication, compassion for oneself, and a readiness to accept change. Selene will discover as she continues reading that she has the ability to not just alter her relationship with exhaustion but also to create a life that exudes vibrancy.

Are you willing to travel with Selene on this adventure? "Energize Your Life" is your compass at this point in time when change is needed. As Selene and each reader find their inner fortitude, let's set out together to leave the darkness of exhaustion behind and enter a life filled with unending energy and fulfillment. Turn the page to start your transformation now.

Understanding Fatigue

A term with more meaning than its letters might suggest is fatigue. It's not merely a passing feeling of fatigue; rather, it's a complicated combination of physical, mental, and emotional components that can overshadow even our best days. To completely overcome fatigue, we must first understand its many facets and disentangle the intricate factors that contribute to its hold.

Categories of Fatigue

The most noticeable type of exhaustion is physical fatigue, which is frequently caused by overexertion, insufficient rest, or physical sickness. It's the heavy sensation in your limbs, the feeling of exhaustion after a long day at work, or the fatigue that follows vigorous exercise.

Mental fatigue: Just like our bodies, our minds may get tired. Mental exhaustion results from prolonged cognitive exertion, multitasking, making decisions, and information processing. It's the cloudy feeling that sets in after hours of intense concentration or the mental fatigue that follows solving challenging issues.

Emotional Fatigue: This kind of exhaustion results from controlling our emotions and juggling social interactions. Stress, lack of empathy, compassion fatigue, and difficult relationships can all contribute to emotional exhaustion. It's that emotional exhaustion that results from putting on a front for others or overcoming obstacles in one's own life. fatigue's root causes

Recognizing the various elements that cause fatigue is necessary for understanding it. Typical causes include:

Lack of Good Sleep: Different forms of Fatigue can be Caused by Lack of Good Sleep or Insufficient Sleep. For both physical and emotional recovery, sleep is essential.

Nutritional Imbalances: Low energy levels and exhaustion can be caused by inadequate nutrition or bad dietary choices.

Chronic Stress: Constantly being under stress without having a good coping method will sap your energy.

Physical health issues: Fatigue can be exacerbated by a number of medical illnesses, including thyroid problems, anemia, and chronic pain.

Mental Health: Anxiety, despair, and burnout are among mental and emotional health issues that can cause weariness.

Overexertion: Fatigue can arise from straining our bodies or minds beyond what they can handle.

Lack of Physical Activity: It's ironic that a sedentary lifestyle can make you feel exhausted.

In order to address each of these elements, we shall investigate tactics and techniques as we delve deeper into the world of weariness. We build the groundwork for a thorough strategy to combat fatigue by comprehending the many forms and causes of exhaustion. information is the first step toward vitality, and armed with this information, we are better able to design a life that escapes the grip of exhaustion.

Discover the methods that will enable you to restore your energy and vitality by turning the page. It's time to solve the riddles of exhaustion and begin living a vibrant, resilient life.

Types of Fatigue

There is no one-size-fits-all definition of fatigue. It shows up in several ways, each with its own nuances and effects. Understanding the various types of weariness will help us better address their underlying causes and customize our coping mechanisms.

Physical Tiredness

The most obvious manifestation of exhaustion is possibly physical fatigue. It's the sensation of bodily weakness, fatigue, and weightiness. This kind of exhaustion frequently results from physically demanding activity, insufficient rest, or extended durations of exertion. Physical tiredness is common among people who work physically demanding jobs, athletes, and manual laborers. However, it can also be brought on by illnesses, ongoing discomfort, or simply pushing oneself past the point of no return.

Mental Tiredness

Long-term cognitive efforts and intensive mental processing are the causes of mental weariness. It's the weariness that follows tasks requiring intense focus, critical thinking, judgment, or problem-solving. Researchers, programmers, and writers are just a few examples of people that commonly feel mental tiredness in their line of work. Reduced focus, slower reaction times, and trouble making decisions are all symptoms of this kind of weariness.

Emotional exhaustion

Managing emotions and navigating social situations lead to emotional exhaustion. People who provide care, work in the medical field, or perform other jobs that demand emotional labor frequently experience emotional tiredness. This kind of exhaustion can be brought on by consistently repressing or controlling emotions, empathizing with others' difficulties, and coping with emotionally charged circumstances that are high-stress. Emotional exhaustion can result in emotional numbness, impatience, and a decreased capacity for interpersonal connection.

Compulsiveness

Compassion fatigue is a distinct subgroup of emotional depletion that affects people in helping professions like therapists, social workers, and first responders who are frequently exposed to the misery and suffering of others. It results from continually providing for others while putting oneself last, leaving one feeling emotionally spent and detached.

Retired

Chronic emotional and physical tiredness known as burnout is a condition that frequently results from long-term exposure to stressful situations and demanding work environments. Cynicism, detachment, and a diminished sense of accomplishment are its defining traits. Work, relationships, and general well-being are just a few of the areas of life that can be affected by burnout.

The first step in dealing with and overcoming these many forms of exhaustion is to comprehend them. Each type calls for particular recuperation and preventative techniques. We can modify our self-care practices, work habits, and lifestyle decisions based on the sort of weariness we're dealing with in order to lessen its effects and recapture our energy and vitality. As we continue on our trip, we'll examine practical solutions to deal with each sort of exhaustion, guiding us toward living a life marked by constant energy and wellbeing.

Causes of Fatigue

The causes of fatigue are frequently complicated interactions between a number of variables, which can make us feel exhausted and depleted. To properly address and manage fatigue, one must have a thorough understanding of its underlying causes. Let's examine a few typical causes:

Lack of Sleep

Inadequate sleep is one of the main causes of weariness. Lack of sleep can make us feel depleted, mentally clouded, and physically exhausted, whether it's because of work obligations, lifestyle decisions, or sleep disorders.

Poor Sleeping Patterns

Even if we get adequate sleep, poor sleep quality might make us feel tired. Sleep disorders such as sleep apnea, insomnia, or restless leg syndrome can interfere with the rejuvenating phases of sleep and keep us from waking up feeling rested.

Nutritional Disproportions

Our energy levels are significantly influenced by our nutrition. Energy crashes and weariness can be brought on by poor nutrition, skipping meals, or ingesting too much processed foods and carbohydrates.

Prolonged Stress

Long-term stress causes the release of stress hormones like cortisol, which over time can cause both physical and mental tiredness. Our energy reserves might be depleted by the body's constant activation of the stress response.

Physical Health Issues

Frustration may be caused by specific medical disorders. Among the problems that can deplete our energy include infections, autoimmune diseases, chronic pain, thyroid abnormalities, anemia, and thyroid disorders.

Issues With Mental Health

Emotional tiredness and general fatigue can result from mental health conditions including anxiety and depression. Both mental and physical health suffer from the ongoing emotional stress.

Sedentary Way of Life

Ironically, not moving around can make you tired. Exercise on a regular basis helps increase vitality, circulation, and energy levels.

Exhaustion

Fatigue might arise from pushing ourselves over our physical or mental limits. Burnout can result from not getting enough rest and recovery time in between periods of exertion.

Dehydration

Weakness can result from even minor dehydration. Water is necessary for many biological processes, including preserving mental and physical vitality.

Pharmaceuticals

Feelings of exhaustion can be exacerbated by some drugs, especially those with sedative effects or those used to treat various medical disorders.

Sugar and Caffeine

Overusing caffeine and sugary meals to get rapid energy boosts can cause energy dumps and eventually make weariness worse.

Poor Psychological and Emotional Health

Mental and emotional exhaustion can be exacerbated by unfavorable emotions, unresolved stress, and a lack of emotional outlets.

Knowing what causes fatigue can help us avoid potential pitfalls and develop effective fatigue management techniques. Addressing the underlying issues is more important than just treating the symptoms. We can reclaim our vitality, vigor, and general well-being by adopting self-care routines, receiving the right medical advice, and making informed lifestyle decisions.

Lifestyle Tips to Boost Your Energy

The appropriate lifestyle choices can make all the difference when it comes to fighting fatigue. You can gradually lay a foundation of constant energy, mental clarity, and general well-being by implementing these techniques into your daily routine. Here are some sensible lifestyle choices to take into account:

Put getting good sleep first.
Establish a regular sleep regimen with a goal of 7-9 hours every night. Establish a relaxing nighttime ritual, avoid using devices right before bed, and maintain a cozy, restful sleeping environment.

Well-Rounded Diet

Feed your body foods that are high in nutrients. Choose a diet that is well-balanced and consists of whole grains, lean proteins, fruits, vegetables, and healthy fats. Avoid refined carbohydrates and excessive sugar, which can cause energy dumps.

Water intake

Stay well hydrated all day long. Drink plenty of water because dehydration might make you feel tired.

Consistent Physical Exercise

Regular exercise will help you feel more energised and fitter overall. Your energy and attitude might benefit from even brief physical activity like walking.

Stress Control

Use stress-reduction methods like yoga, meditation, deep breathing, or mindfulness. Effective stress management can stop the onset of chronic fatigue.

Work-Life Harmony

Set limits between your personal and professional lives. Give yourself time to unwind, indulge in your interests, and spend quality time with your loved ones.

Time Management That Works

To avoid burnout and preserve productivity, prioritize work, break your day into small chunks, and take regular breaks.

Nutritious Snacks

Choose snacks that are well-balanced and contain protein, fiber, and healthy fats. These snacks might offer steady energy levels all day long.

Social Relationship

Maintain social connections and meaningful partnerships. Your mental health can be improved by spending time with loved ones and participating in constructive interactions.

Relaxation and mindfulness

Add relaxation and mindfulness exercises to your daily routine. Deep breathing, progressive muscle relaxation, and guided imagery are all effective ways to relax and reduce stress.

Enough rest and recuperation

When engaging in physically demanding activities, especially, pay attention to your body and give it time to rest and recover. Give yourself permission to rest since overworking yourself might make you tired.

Consult a professional

Consider talking to a healthcare provider if your fatigue continues despite using these measures. Your weariness may be a result of underlying medical issues or nutritional deficits.

Keep in mind that overcoming exhaustion is a long process that calls for patience and consistency. Start by integrating one or two of these lifestyle choices into your daily routine, then add more over time. As you put these changes into practice, pay attention to how your body reacts and make adjustments as necessary. You can recover your energy and vitality with commitment and a holistic approach, enabling you to flourish in every area of your life.

Sleep and relaxation: refuel for energy

Sleep and rest frequently take a backseat to our commitments and responsibilities in our fast-paced life. But ignoring these vital components of wellbeing might make us tired, impair our cognitive abilities, and even jeopardize our general health. Let's examine the relevance of rest and sleep as well as ways to maximize them for a life that is full of vigor and energy.

The Value of a Good Night's Sleep

Sleep is a critical physiological process that renews our body and mind, not just a moment of idleness. Our brain consolidates memories, manages emotions, and maintains cognitive activities when we sleep. Additionally, it's a time for immune system boosting, hormone balancing, and tissue repair. Sleeping enough is important for:

Restoring Energy: A restful night's sleep replenishes our energy stores, enabling us to take on the day with vigor. Our capacity to think, learn, solve issues, and make judgments is improved by sleep.

Emotional Well-Being: A restful night's sleep supports emotional stability.
Physical Well-Being: Sleep promotes immunity, cardiovascular health, and

metabolism- and appetite-regulating hormones-regulation.

Techniques for Getting More Rest

Schedule Consistency: Even on weekends, establish a consistent sleep schedule by going to bed and waking up at the same times every day.
Establishing a calming bedtime routine Before going to bed, practice relaxation techniques like reading, doing some light stretching, or listening to relaxing music.

Environment Awareness Keep a peaceful, calm, and dark environment for sleeping.

Consider using blackout curtains and lowering noise interference.

Limit Your Screen Time: Screens (phones, tablets, and computers) should be avoided at least an hour before bed since the blue light they emit can interfere with the hormones that make you fall asleep.

Reduce Stimulants: Avoid caffeine and large meals right before night because they can interfere with your sleep.

Manage Stress: To help calm your thoughts before sleeping, try relaxation techniques like deep breathing or meditation.

Limiting naps is a good idea because extended naps throughout the day can disrupt your ability to sleep at night, even though short naps can be revitalizing.

Exercise: Getting regular exercise will help you sleep better, but try to avoid doing an intensive workout just before bed.

Adopt Relaxing Activities

Rest includes planned rest throughout the day and is not only confined to sleep. You can refuel and prevent fatigue from building up by participating in relaxing activities. Consider:

Utilize brief breaks during your working day to stretch, get up and walk around, and clear your head.

Moments of Mindfulness: To center oneself and lower stress throughout the day, practice mindfulness or deep breathing techniques.

Hobbies: Make time for the pursuit of your interests, whether they be leisure pursuits like reading, gardening, or painting.

Spend time outside and make a connection with nature to reenergize your senses and unclutter your mind.

Your energy levels and general well-being can be greatly affected by prioritizing good sleep and embracing downtime. Your path to maintained vigor and a more contented existence is paved with the development of healthy sleeping patterns and the regular practice of relaxing activities. Never forget that getting enough sleep and rest is an important investment in your wellbeing.

Providing Energy Through Nutrition and Hydration

Our energy levels, cognitive ability, and general well-being are significantly influenced by the meals we eat and the fluids we drink. The keys to overcoming weariness and keeping a robust life are proper nutrition and hydration. Let's discuss methods to maximize your diet and hydration for long-lasting energy as well as the significance of feeding your body.

The Function of Nutrition

Our bodies' essential building blocks are provided by nutrition. A diet that is well-balanced guarantees a consistent supply of the nutrients needed for physical and mental health, as well as for the creation of energy. Important vitamins and minerals that support vitality include:

Carbohydrates are the body's main energy source and fuel for both mental and physical activity.

Proteins: Crucial for immune system health, tissue repair, and preserving muscular mass. Include plant-based protein sources, lean meats, fish, beans, and fish.

Fats are essential for the health of the brain and the storage of energy. Consider fatty fish, nuts, seeds, and avocados as your sources.

Vitamins and minerals: These micronutrients are essential for a number of biological processes, such as the creation of energy and the maintenance of the immune system.

All biological processes, such as digestion, circulation, and temperature regulation, depend on water for proper function.

Optimal Nutrition Techniques

Meals that are well-balanced should have a range of ingredients, such as lean proteins, healthy grains, vibrant fruits, and vegetables.

Regular Meals: In order to keep your energy levels consistent throughout the day, try to eat at regular intervals. Do not miss meals.

Mindful Snacking: To keep your energy levels up between meals, choose nutrient-dense snacks that mix protein, fiber, and healthy fats.

Make sure you're well hydrated by sipping lots of water throughout the day. To encourage frequent sips, keep a reusable water bottle with you.

Limit processed and sugary foods: Limit processed foods and sugary snacks because they might cause energy crashes.

Containment Portions: To prevent overeating and guarantee a balanced diet, pay close attention to portion proportions.

Prioritize fiber: To aid with digestion and control energy release, include fiber-rich foods such as whole grains, legumes, fruits, and vegetables.

Limit your intake of alcohol and caffeine, which, while they may momentarily boost your mood or give you more energy, can also disrupt your sleep and cause erratic energy levels.

The Influence of Hydration

For the maintenance of energy levels, cognitive function, and general wellness, staying properly hydrated is crucial. Dehydration can result in weariness and lowered cognitive function. Even if you don't feel thirsty, make an effort to drink water frequently during the day.

Adopt Mindful Eating

By paying attention to your body's signals of hunger and fullness, you can practice mindful eating. Enjoy the taste of your food by chewing carefully. To truly enjoy your meals and minimize overeating, stay away from distractions when eating, such as devices.

Look for Expert Advice

For individualized advice on your nutritional requirements and any particular health problems you may have, think about consulting a qualified dietitian or nutritionist.

You're giving your body the building blocks it needs for vitality by making wise food choices and putting hydration first. You can approach each day with renewed vigor and enthusiasm if you consume the right foods, drink the right amounts of water, and maintain a healthy weight.

Energize Your Life with Exercise and Physical Activity

Exercise is a great way to fight weariness, improve mood, and improve general wellbeing in addition to keeping healthy. Regular exercise can assist you in escaping the grip of exhaustion and bringing new vitality into your life. Examining the value of exercise and how to fit it into your daily routine will help you maintain your vigor.

The Advantages of Exercise

Beyond improving physical health, regular exercise has a host of other advantages. Your energy levels, general quality of life, and mental and emotional health are all significantly impacted. Exercise has many advantages, such as:

Increased Energy: Physical activity boosts blood flow and oxygen delivery, which might help you feel more energised and fight weariness.

Better Mood: Exercise triggers the release of endorphins, or "feel-good" hormones, which can improve your mood and lower stress.

Improved Sleep: Exercise on a regular basis can help regulate your sleep cycles, resulting in better sleep and greater alertness during the day.

Benefits for the Mind: Exercise has been linked to better cognitive function, including better focus, memory, and problem-solving skills.

Exercise offers a healthy way to release stress and lessen the development of tension in your body.

Techniques to Include Physical Activity

Choose Activities You Truly Enjoy, Whether It's Walking, Jogging, Dancing, Swimming, Cycling, or Playing Sports, Find Activities You Truly Enjoy.

Start Slowly: If you've never exercised before, start out easy and gradually increase your duration and intensity.

Realistic Goal Setting To stay motivated, set reasonable exercise objectives. Along the journey, recognize your accomplishments.

Create a routine: Like any other appointment, schedule frequent fitness sessions. Gaining the advantages of exercise requires consistency.

Combining cardiovascular and strength training exercises will result in a well-rounded fitness regimen. Examples of cardiovascular exercises include walking, jogging, cycling, and weightlifting.

Break it Up: If you are unable to dedicate a substantial amount of time to exercise, divide it up into smaller sessions spread out throughout the day.

Exercise as a Way to Socialize: To turn physical activity into a social experience, join a sports league, a group fitness class, or an exercise club.

Observe Your Body: Consider how your body reacts to activity. To avoid becoming exhausted or burned out, take time to rest when you need to.

Mind-Body Exercises: Yoga, Pilates, tai chi, and other mind-body exercises are good options. Along with improving flexibility and balance, these activities also encourage unwinding and stress relief.

Adopt a holistic viewpoint: Keep in mind that exercise is only one component of a comprehensive plan. For overall wellness, combine regular physical activity with a healthy diet, plenty of water, and enough sleep.

You're investing in your physical and mental health by making exercise a part of your daily routine. Every action you take, whether it's a morning jog, a dance class, or a leisurely stroll, moves you one step closer to living a life that is brimming with vitality, optimism, and a sense of success. Use exercise as a tool to combat exhaustion and embrace a life that is vibrant.

Navigating Calmness in Stress Management

In a world full with obligations and demands, stress may be a constant companion, draining your energy and making you exhausted. Maintaining your general wellbeing and preventing weariness requires effective stress management. Let's discuss the significance of stress management and methods for cultivating serenity in the face of difficulties.

Understanding Stress

Your body's reaction to perceived threats or challenges is stress. Chronic stress can result in physical and emotional weariness, although short-term stress can be stimulating. Unmanaged stress can affect your physical health as well as cause exhaustion and mood swings.

The Influence of Stress Reduction

Adopting strategies and routines that support a healthy response to stressors is essential for stress management. You may lessen the negative effects chronic stress has on your well-being and energy levels by doing this. Among the advantages of stress management are:

Increased Energy: Stress management guards against the depleting effects of persistent stress on your body and mind.

Enhanced Coping: Stress management gives you the tools you need to face problems with emotional stability and resilience.

Better Sleep: Stress management practices can enhance the quality of sleep, which raises energy levels during the day.

Emotional Health: Stress management can lessen or even eliminate the signs of anxiety and sadness.

Effective Stress Management Techniques

Meditation and mindfulness exercises can help you stay present and lower your stress levels. These methods promote relaxation and improve your capacity for stress management.

Exercises involving deep breathing can help you reduce tension and trigger your body's relaxation response.

Exercise on a regular basis: Exercise naturally lowers stress. Exercise results in the release of the hormones endorphins, which elevate mood.

Management of time: Make a realistic timetable and order your tasks according to importance to avoid feeling overburdened by your obligations.

Lean on your friends, family, or support networks while you're under stress.

Seeking counsel and talking about your feelings can help you feel better.

Hobbies and Creative Outlets: Taking part in activities you enjoy, such as gardening, playing an instrument, or painting, might help you focus on something else while dealing with stress.

Healthy Boundaries: Establish boundaries to stop yourself from going overboard. To avoid unnecessary stress, learn to say no when it is essential.

Challenge negative thoughts and replace them with positive affirmations by engaging in positive self-talk. You can increase your outlook and resiliency by using positive self-talk.

Relaxation Techniques: Use techniques to help you unwind, such as progressive muscle relaxation or guided visualization.

Seek Professional Assistance: If stress becomes unbearable or persistent, you might want to go to a therapist or counselor.

Develop Mindful Moments: Include small mindfulness breaks throughout the day. These thoughtful breaks can assist you in controlling stress and regaining attention, whether they consist of a few deep breaths, a little walk, or a quiet moment of reflection.

Your Way to Calmness: The goal of stress management is to give yourself the tools to properly handle stress, not to completely eradicate it. Adopting stress management techniques is a proactive step towards restoring your energy, achieving emotional equilibrium, and building a resilient, peaceful existence.

Regaining Restful Nights: Improving Sleep Quality

The foundation of vigor and wellbeing is good sleep. Focusing on enhancing your sleep quality can make a world of difference if you frequently struggle with weariness and restlessness. Explore the importance of good sleep quality and learn how to establish a setting that promotes restful evenings and reviving sleep.

The significance of good sleep: How well you sleep at night is referred to as your sleep quality. It's important to have quality, restorative sleep in addition to getting enough sleep. No matter how long you've been in bed, getting poor quality sleep can make you feel sleepy, cranky, and exhausted during the day.

Techniques to Improve Sleep Quality: Create a Consistent Routine: Even on weekends, go to bed and get up at the same times every day. Your body's internal clock can be regulated through consistency.

Make Your Sleep Environment Comfortable: Your sleeping space should promote relaxation. Maintain a calm, quiet, and dark environment to encourage restful sleep.

Avoid using screens right before bed: A hormone that controls sleep, melatonin, can't be produced by your body properly when exposed to the blue light that screens emit. At least an hour before bedtime, stay away from devices.

Relaxation Exercise: Create a relaxing nighttime ritual. Reading, light stretching, or meditation might help your body know when it's time to wind down.

Avoid consuming heavy, spicy, or caffeine-containing foods right before bed. These could make it difficult to sleep or make you uncomfortable at night.

Keep Moving During the Day: Regular exercise can enhance sleep quality, but avoid strenuous activities right before bed.

Limiting naps is a good idea because they can disrupt nocturnal sleep, even if brief naps can be revitalizing.

Manage Stress: To relax your mind before bed, try stress-reduction exercises like deep breathing or meditation.
A solid mattress and soft pillows can significantly improve the quality of your sleep.

Avoid alcohol and nicotine because they can interfere with your sleep and make it less restful.

Regulate Light Exposure: You can aid your body's internal clock by exposing yourself to natural light during the day and low lighting at night.

Rituals for a Good Night's Sleep: Make relaxing activities a part of your nighttime routine. Take part in relaxing activities, such drinking herbal tea, reading a book, or taking a warm bath.

The Path to a Good Night's Sleep: The quest to better sleep quality calls for persistence and dedication. Try out different combinations of these tactics to see which suits you the best. Setting a high priority on getting quality sleep may completely change your days, giving them increased vigor, focus, and well-being. Keep in mind that getting enough sleep each night helps you stay strong and healthy overall.

Hygiene Advice for Sleep

Adopting healthy routines and procedures that encourage sound sleep is known as sleep hygiene. You may foster a setting that supports restful sleep by implementing these suggestions into your daily routine. Let's look at some important sleep hygiene advice so you may reclaim your nights and wake up feeling rejuvenated.

Keep a Regular Sleep Schedule: Even on weekends, go to bed and get up at the same hours every day. Your body's internal clock can be regulated through consistency.

Establish a relaxing sleeping environment:
Your bedroom should be cold, quiet, and dark. To create the optimal sleeping environment, think about utilizing blackout curtains, earplugs, or a white noise machine.

Limit your evening screen time: At least an hour before going to bed, stay away from displays (phones, tablets, computers). The generation of melatonin by your body may be hampered by the blue light that screens emit.

Create a Calming Bedtime Schedule: Before going to bed, practice relaxing activities like reading, light stretching, meditation, or deep breathing.

Watch What You Eat: Avoid consuming coffee, alcohol, or large or heavy meals right before bed. These may make it difficult to sleep or make you uncomfortable at night.

Keep Moving Throughout the Day: Regular exercise can enhance the quality of your sleep, but try to finish your workout before bed.

Limiting naps: Long naps that could disrupt your overnight sleep should be avoided, even though they might be refreshing during the day.

Control Stress: To help you relax before bed, practice stress-reduction methods during the day, such as yoga, meditation, or mindfulness.

Control the Exposure to Light: To improve your body's internal clock, spend time in natural light during the day and decrease the lights at night.

Make Your Bedding Comfortable: For healthy sleep, make sure your mattress and pillows offer sufficient support and comfort.

Save your bed for intimacy and sleep: Avoid doing things like working or watching TV on your bed. Your mind will more readily identify your bed as a place of rest if you associate it with sleep.

Keep an eye on fluid intake: Drink plenty of water during the day, but cut back on it in the hours before bed to avoid waking up to use the restroom.

Relax before bed: As part of your evening ritual, do something calming. Your body will receive this signal that it is time to get ready for sleep.

If Professional Assistance Is Needed: Consider seeking advice from a healthcare expert if, despite following excellent sleep hygiene, you still have trouble falling asleep.

A Regular Routine: Keep in mind that practicing excellent sleep hygiene requires consistency. Gradually put these suggestions into practice and experiment to see what works best for you. These behaviors over time can improve the quality of your sleep, enabling you to wake up rested and prepared to take on the day with renewed vigor and focus.

Establishing a Calming Bedtime Routine: De-stress and Get Ready for Sleep

A relaxing nighttime routine that tells your body it's time to wind down can greatly enhance the quality of your sleep. This step-by-step tutorial will show you how to establish a relaxing bedtime routine that will help you go from the pressures of the day to a sound night's sleep.

Establish a Regular Bedtime: Set a fixed time each night to begin your nighttime ritual. Your body's internal clock can be regulated through consistency.

Dim the Lighting: Dimmer the lights in your living area to start. Your body will receive a signal from this that it is time to get ready for sleep.

Disconnect your screens: At least an hour before going to bed, turn off all electronic devices, including phones, tablets, and computers. The generation of melatonin by your body may be hampered by the blue light that screens emit.

Take a Warm Shower or Bath: Warm baths or showers can ease tense muscles and clear the mind. Warm water's calming effect can be a good way to induce sleep.

Practice Yoga or gentle stretching: Consider adding some light stretching or a quick yoga practice to your routine. Concentrate on stretching your body gently to relieve stress.

Take up meditation or deep breathing exercises: Practice deep breathing techniques or engage in a brief period of meditation. This can assist in stress reduction and mental calmness.

Spend Time Reading or Listening to Calm Music: It might be relaxing to unwind by reading a tranquil book or listening to relaxing music. Pick furnishings and decor that put you at ease and relaxation.

Drink Herbal Tea: Have a cup of herbal tea without caffeine, like chamomile or valerian root tea. These teas may help you wind down before night and promote relaxation.

Keep a journal: Write down your thoughts, reflections, or things for which you are grateful in a journal for a short while. This can aid in mind-clearing before bed.

Establish a Relaxing Sleep Environment: When you're prepared to sleep, make sure your bedroom is a cozy and tranquil setting. Make the room cooler and the lights even dimmer as you like.

Limit Your Fluid Intake: Reduce your fluid consumption in the evening to prevent nighttime awakenings due to restroom trips.

Show gratitude: Take a time before going to bed to think back on your day's highlights and be thankful for them.

Employ relaxation methods: To further relax your body and mind, incorporate relaxation techniques such as progressive muscle relaxation or guided visualization.

Keep Being Consistent

Maintain a consistent nighttime routine. Your body will eventually come to link these relaxing activities with falling asleep.

Creating Your Individual Schedule

You are welcome to modify this program to fit your tastes and way of life. The secret is to do things that will help you relax and make the transition from a busy day to a quiet night of sleep easy. By maintaining a regular and relaxing nighttime routine, you're creating the conditions for restful sleep that leaves you feeling revived and energised the next day.

Managing Sleep Disorders: Reclaiming Restful Nights

To enhance your sleep quality and general wellbeing if you have a sleep issue, it's critical to have a good diagnosis and therapy. Consulting a healthcare practitioner is essential because different sleep disorders call for different treatment methods. Here is a general outline of how to treat frequent sleep disorders:

Insomnia

Inability to get to sleep, stay asleep, or have restorative sleep while having enough opportunity.

Management:

Set up a regular sleeping pattern.

Establish a peaceful bedtime routine.

Reduce your intake of alcohol and caffeine, especially in the evening.

Keep your bedroom quiet, dark, and cozy.

Take into account cognitive-behavioral therapy (CBT) for insomnia, which focuses on altering beliefs and actions that cause sleep issues.

Snoring Apnea

Breathing repeatedly stops and begins while you're sleeping, disrupting your sleep and even putting your health in danger.

Management: For a diagnosis and possible treatments, speak with a medical expert.

For obstructive sleep apnea, continuous positive airway pressure (CPAP) therapy is a frequent treatment.

A change in lifestyle, such as losing weight and abstaining from alcohol before night, can also aid in the management of sleep apnea.

RLS (Restless Legs Syndrome):

An uncontrollable impulse to move one's legs as a result of unpleasant feelings, which frequently get worse while one is at rest or inactive.

Management: To ensure a correct diagnosis, speak with a medical practitioner.

Find and stay away from triggers that exacerbate symptoms.

To manage the stress caused by RLS, practice stress-reduction methods.

RLS symptoms can be effectively managed with medications and lifestyle modifications.

Narcolepsy

A neurological condition that causes irregular sleep patterns, extreme daytime sleepiness, and sudden loss of muscular tone (cataplexy).

Management: For a diagnosis and possible treatments, speak with a medical expert.

Symptoms can be managed with the aid of medications and lifestyle changes.

Set a regular bedtime and give proper sleep hygiene a high priority.

RBD, or REM sleep behavior disorder

Definition: A condition when a person plays out vivid dreams physically while they are in REM sleep, frequently causing harm to themselves or their sleeping partner.

Management: For a diagnosis and possible treatments, speak with a medical expert.

Safety precautions, such as eliminating potentially harmful objects from the sleeping area, are essential.

RBD symptoms can be managed with the aid of medications and behavioral treatments.

Getting Professional Assistance

It's crucial to speak with a medical professional, such as a sleep specialist or a physician with experience in sleep medicine, about any sleep disturbance. They are able to correctly identify the illness and suggest the best courses of action or therapy for your particular needs. If you're having trouble sleeping, don't be afraid to get treatment; correctly managing sleep disorders can greatly enhance your quality of life and general health.

Embracing Vitality from Morning to Night: Energizing Your Day

It takes a holistic strategy that integrates several facets of your lifestyle to start the day with energy and keep it throughout the day. Here is a strategy to help you start your day off well and keep it that way all day long.

Morning:

Get up early to get your day going. Set a regular wake-up time. This encourages better-quality sleep by regulating your body's internal schedule.

Hydrate: After a long night of sleep, start your day with a glass of water to rehydrate your body and jump-start your metabolism.

Healthy Breakfast: Start your day off right with a protein-, whole-grain-, and fruit or vegetable-rich breakfast.

Morning Exercise: Move your body gently to stimulate blood flow in the morning. Examples of this include stretching or a quick walk.

Practice mindfulness to set a good mood for the day by devoting a few minutes to it, deep breathing, or meditation.

Daytime:

Keep Hydrated: To sustain your energy levels and support bodily functions, drink water throughout the day.

Healthy Snacking: To maintain your energy between meals, choose nutrient-dense snacks that contain protein, fiber, and healthy fats.
Take frequent breaks to stretch, walk around, and relax your thoughts while your work or daily tasks.

Lunch that is Nutrient-Rich: To maintain a stable level of energy, choose a lunch that is well-balanced and contains lean proteins, veggies, and whole grains.

Stay Active: Try to fit in brief bouts of exercise throughout the day, such as walking quickly or using the stairs.

Evening:
Eat mindfully by having a light, balanced dinner that won't make you feel stuffed before night.

Limit Screen Time: Limit your evening screen time to give your body time to unwind and get ready for bed.

Read a book, listen to some relaxing music, or take a warm bath as examples of relaxing hobbies.

Unplug: To avoid exposure to blue light, which can interfere with sleep, put away electronic gadgets at least an hour before bed.

Sleep hygiene: Establish a regular bedtime routine that encourages sound sleep. Prioritize proper sleep hygiene routines and create a comfortable sleeping environment.

Overall:

Balanced nutrition involves consuming nutrient-dense foods that give you long-lasting energy and promote your general health.

Regular Physical Activity: Include regular physical activity in your routine to improve mood and increase energy. Practice stress-reduction strategies to avoid emotional and mental depletion. Stress management.

Drink enough of water throughout the day to preserve your energy and cognitive performance.
Take mindful breaks throughout the day to reconnect with the present and lower your stress levels.

You're establishing a lifestyle that encourages continuous energy and vigor from morning to night by incorporating these routines into your daily schedule. Keep in mind that even seemingly insignificant adjustments can have a big impact on your day-to-day mood and ultimately contribute to a more vivid and satisfying existence.

Energize Your Day from the Start with Morning Routines

A well-designed morning routine can help you start the day with vigor and purpose and create a favorable tone for the remainder of the day. Here are some tips for creating a morning routine that can energize your body, mind, and spirit.

Arrive Early

Set a regular wake-up time to start your day. This creates a sense of habit and aids in regulating your body's internal clock.

Hydration

After several hours of sleep, start with drinking a glass of water to rehydrate your body. Squeeze some lemon juice in for an additional bit of coolness.

Consciousness Training

Give mindfulness, meditation, or deep breathing some time. Set a good tone for the day by making them.

Morning Activity

Do some light exercise to get your blood circulating. Stretching, brisk walking, or a brief yoga session can all be used for this.

Wholesome breakfast

A healthy breakfast that combines protein, whole grains, and fruits or vegetables will fuel your body. Avoid sweet foods that could cause energy dumps.

Set Important Tasks in Priority

Take on your most crucial chores or initiatives first thing in the morning. You'll have a sense of accomplishment and start the day off productively.

Check Your Goals

Review your daily objectives for a moment. This keeps you motivated and concentrated all day long.

Disconnect from screens

To minimize distractions and give your mind a chance to properly awaken in the morning, limit your screen time.

Affirmations of the positive

Use affirmations and self-talk that is constructive. Consider your capabilities and skills for the day.

Think ahead

Establish your goals for the day and make a to-do list. Knowing what has to be done might help you stay organized and reduce stress.

Get in touch with loved ones

Spend some time talking to your housemates, family, or pets. Having pleasant interactions might improve your mood.

Get ready for the day:

Prepare oneself by grooming, selecting a clothes, and gathering the day's necessities. Having a polished appearance might increase your confidence.

Affirm your gratitude

Give thanks for the new day and the opportunity it provides for a minute.

Be consistent

Consistency is the key to a productive morning routine. To benefit, try to follow a similar schedule every day.

Make adjustments to your morning routine based on your tastes and way of living. The objective is to plan a series of activities that will excite and inspire you for the upcoming day. Remember that a productive morning routine can set the tone for your entire day and lead to a more contented and successful existence.

Nutritious Snacking for Long-Lasting Energy: Thrive

The appropriate snacks can give you constant energy throughout the day, preventing energy crashes and enabling you to maintain concentrate. Here is a guide on choosing wholesome snacks that will fuel your body and maintain a constant level of energy.

Add Macronutrients Together: Choose snacks that combine healthy fats, carbohydrates, and proteins. Long-lasting energy is produced and blood sugar levels are stabilized by this equilibrium.

Select Whole Foods: Keep your attention on whole, minimally processed foods. Whole grains, nuts, seeds, and fresh produce are all healthy options.

Think ahead: To prevent reaching for bad foods when you're hungry, make snacks in advance.

Portion Regulation: To avoid overeating and to ensure a balanced intake of nutrients, pay attention to portion sizes.

Healthy Alternatives: Choose healthy snacks that are high in vitamins, minerals, and antioxidants. These consist of nuts, fruits, and vegetables.

Foods High in Fiber: Pick fiber-rich snacks to help you feel full and to give you long-lasting energy. Apples, carrots, and whole grain crackers are some examples.

Contains Protein Snacks: Protein serves as a slow-release energy source and keeps you feeling full. Lean turkey slices, Greek yogurt, and cottage cheese are all excellent sources of protein.

Suitable Fats: Include healthy fats from nuts, seeds, and avocados in your diet. These fats improve general wellness and offer steady energy.

Nut Butter Treats: For a filling and energizing snack, combine nut butters (peanut, almond, or cashew) with whole grain crackers, apple slices, or celery.

Energy Snacks: Utilizing oats, nuts, seeds, and dried fruits, you can make your own energy snacks. These portable snacks are nutrient-dense and simple to make.

Parfait of Greek yogurt: Greek yogurt, fresh fruit, and honey are combined to make a delightful and high-protein snack.

Veggies and hummus: For a filling and nutrient-rich snack, dunk colorful veggie sticks in hummus.

Path Mix: Make your own trail mix with a combination of nuts, seeds, dried fruits, and a trace of dark chocolate for a treat that will give you more energy.

Water Quality Matters: Consider drinking water along with your snacks to stay hydrated. Feelings of exhaustion may result from dehydration.

Observe your body: Pay attention to your hunger signals and select snacks that satiate your appetites and provide you with the energy you need.

102

Snacking on healthy foods is crucial to sustaining constant energy levels throughout the day. You may give your body the energy it needs to thrive, stay focused, and carry out your daily chores with vigor by choosing nutrient-dense, balanced snacks.

Emotional and Mental Health

In order to stay healthy and vital overall, it's important to take care of your mental and emotional wellbeing. Here is a guide to developing a happy outlook and caring for your mental wellbeing.

Engage in Self-Care: Give the things that make you happy and relaxed top priority. Take up a hobby, go outside for a while, or just relax for a while.

Meditation and mindfulness: Include mindfulness exercises in your daily routine. Deep breathing, mindfulness, and meditation can all support emotional balance and stress management.

Positivity in Oneself: Positive affirmations should take the place of negative ones. Develop self-compassion and gentleness toward oneself.

Seek Assistance: When you need to talk, reach out to friends, family, or experts. A sense of comfort and perspective might come from sharing your feelings.

Establish Limits: To safeguard your mental and emotional well-being, set healthy boundaries. Recognize when you should say no.

Possess gratitude: Think about the things you have to be thankful for often. Exercises that focus on gratitude can improve your attitude and help you see the good things in life.

Associated with Others: Create and maintain important connections. A sense of belonging and emotional support are provided through social bonds.

Reduce Stress: To avoid burnout and overwhelm, use stress-reduction strategies including exercise, relaxation, and time management.

Be able to let go: Accept what you cannot change and concentrate your efforts on influencing the things you can. Perfectionism can increase stress, so let go of it.

Develop Your Resilience: Develop the capacity to overcome obstacles. Consider setbacks as chances for development and education.

Expression of Emotion: Give yourself permission to let your emotions out in healthy ways. You can process and control your feelings with the aid of writing, art, and conversation.

Putting sleep first: Sleep is essential for maintaining emotional health. Create a cozy sleeping environment and establish a regular sleep schedule.

Take Part in Activities You Enjoy: Spend time engaging in activities that bring you joy and fulfillment. Hobbies increase your sense of fulfillment and purpose.

Reduce Screen Time: Set limits on screen time to avoid overexposure to stressful social media and negative news.

Get Professional Assistance: If you experience ongoing emotional difficulties, you might want to think about getting help from a mental health expert.

Keeping in mind that mental and emotional health is a process. The key to developing a happy and balanced mentality that promotes your general vitality and quality of life is to prioritize self-care, manage stress, and nurture your emotional wellbeing.

Finding inner peace using mindfulness and relaxation techniques

You may manage stress, improve focus, and support emotional wellbeing by using mindfulness and relaxation techniques. Here is a roadmap to adding these habits to your daily schedule.

Conscious Breathing: Observe your breathing. Slowly take a four-count inhalation, then take a four-count exhalation. You can become present with the help of this straightforward technique.

Meditation using Body Scan: Sit or lie down comfortably. Gradually turn your focus to every bodily part, observing sensations without passing judgment.

Directed Imagery: Close your eyes and picture a serene setting. Consider what you can see, hear, and smell. Take full advantage of this mental retreat.

Progressively relaxing the muscles: Starting at your toes and working your way up, tense and then relax each muscle group. This method relieves stress in the body.

Conscious Eating: Each bite you eat should be thoroughly enjoyed in terms of flavor, texture, and scent. This method encourages mindful eating and enjoyment.

Grounding Procedures: To help you stay in the present, use your senses. Count the number of senses you can use: five items you can see, four you can touch, three you can hear, two you can smell, and one you can taste.

Observant Walking: Walk while paying attention to each stride. Pay attention to the sound of your breath and the feel of the ground beneath your feet.

Self-Compassion Meditation: Send yourself, your loved ones, and even people you might disagree with, sentiments of love and compassion.

Deep Inhalation: Breathe in deeply for a count of four through your nose, hold for a count of four, and then exhale through your mouth for a count of six. Several times, repeat.

Reflective journaling: Without passing judgment, jot down your feelings and thoughts. Think back on your experiences, then try to be grateful.

Nature Relationship: Spend time in nature by being outside. Be mindful of the sights, sounds, and textures that are all around you.

Electronic detox: Take pauses from using electronics. Disconnecting from devices can ease stress and create mental space.

Peaceful Music: Listen to relaxing music to help you relax and calm your mind.

Visualization: Imagine yourself in a serene, safe environment. To facilitate a mental getaway, visualize every aspect.

Keep your attention on the here and now, whatever you're doing. To truly immerse yourself in the event, use all of your senses.

Add these mindfulness and relaxation exercises as needed to your routine. You may build emotional wellbeing, reduce stress, and improve your everyday life's sense of serenity and balance with regular practice.

Work-life harmony: juggling work and personal obligations

Maintaining overall wellbeing and avoiding burnout require finding a balance between work and personal life. Here is a handbook to assist you in balancing your personal demands and work obligations.

Establish Limits: Establish distinct lines separating work and leisure time. Do not answer calls or check work emails after hours.

Put self-care first: Make taking care of yourself a priority in your daily routine. Take part in physical, mental, and emotional recharging activities.

Plan & Prepare: To manage your projects and set aside time for both business and personal activities, use calendars and to-do lists.

Management of time: Use time management techniques. Set priorities for your work, assign duties when you can, and refrain from taking on too many commitments.
Say no more often.

Before beginning a new task, evaluate your capacity. Saying no when it's necessary enables you to safeguard your time and energy.

Unplug: Set aside time each day to turn off all work-related devices and activities. Give yourself permission to completely engage in private moments.

Make Your Workspace Productive: Organize your workspace to maximize productivity. An orderly environment might make it easier for you to perform chores.

Plan your leisure time: Make time for your favorite hobbies outside of work. Schedule leisure activities, exercise, socializing, and downtime.

Delegate and Enlist Assistance: Don't be afraid to ask relatives and friends for help with personal obligations or to outsource jobs at work.

Aware Transitions: Apply mindfulness practices when switching between your personal and professional lives. To refocus, take a few deep breaths.

Flexibility: Be flexible with your schedule. Being adaptive aids in keeping a healthy balance because life can be unpredictable.

Superior Quality to Quantity: Instead of concentrating on the quantity, think about the quality of your interactions and work. Quality increases satisfaction.

Take a Lesson Every Day: Think about your regular activities. Decide which components of your duty balance worked well and which could use improvement.

Set realistic objectives: Set realistic objectives for your personal and professional lives. Unneeded stress might result from having unrealistic expectations.

Interaction: Tell your coworkers, family, and friends about your boundaries and needs. Open dialogue promotes comprehension.

Keep in mind that finding balance is a process that may require changes along the way. Living a more contented and peaceful existence is made possible by placing equal importance on your work and personal well-being.

Increasing Your Network of Support and Connections for Your Well-Being

Maintaining your mental and emotional well-being fundamentally involves asking for help and building relationships with others. Here are some tips for getting help and making deep connections:

Understand the Importance: Recognize that asking for help does not indicate weakness but rather power. A network of supporters is useful for everyone.

Speak with family and friends: Share your ideas and feelings with those you love. Sometimes, getting things off your chest by simply talking about them.

Have In-Depth Conversations: Start conversations that are more in-depth than idle chatter. Talk openly and honestly about your feelings, opinions, and experiences with individuals you trust.

Participate in Helpful Communities: Become a part of organizations, clubs, or online communities that share your interests or objectives. Finding others who share your interests can help you feel like you belong.

Look for Expert Assistance: Consider speaking with a therapist, counselor, or mental health specialist if you're facing serious difficulties.

Continual Interaction: Maintain open lines of communication with your loved ones. Encourage them to do the same by clearly stating your demands and boundaries.

Develop Empathy: Practice empathy by paying close attention when others are sharing their stories and demonstrating understanding.

Attend social gatherings: Engage in social activities that you find appealing.

These gatherings can offer chances to network and meet new individuals.

Volunteer: You can meet people who share your interests and feel fulfilled by volunteering.

Reestablish contact with old friends: Make contact with any friends you may have forgotten about. Making old ties again might be fruitful.

Internet networking: Use social media to reach out to old friends, meet new people, and have insightful conversations.

Advocacy Groups: Consider joining a group of people going through like difficulties. These groups provide a secure setting for communication and comprehension.

Use active listening techniques: When others express their feelings, pay close attention to what they are saying. Relationships can be strengthened by lending a sympathetic ear.

Participate in seminars and workshops: Attend conferences, seminars, and workshops that are relevant to your interests. These gatherings offer chances for networking and education.

Be Present

Be completely in the present when interacting with others. Give people your whole attention and participate in sincere dialogue.

Developing a strong support system and looking for meaningful relationships can have a big impact on your mental and emotional health. Keep in mind that developing relationships takes time, and maintaining those ties takes work. You may develop a network that enhances your life if you have an open mind and are eager to participate.

Time management and output

A more happy and balanced existence can be attained by efficiently managing your time and enhancing productivity. Here is a guide to help you make the most of your time, achieve your objectives, and stay healthy.

Define Specific Goals: Set both immediate and long-term objectives. Your responsibilities and priorities will be guided by your sense of purpose.

Set task priorities: Identify the day's most crucial duties. Put jobs into categories based on their relevance and urgency using tools like the Eisenhower Matrix.

Compile a list of tasks: In a to-do list, note tasks, due dates, and commitments. This helps you stay organized and stops things from getting overlooked.

Utilize time blocking: Set up distinct time periods for various tasks. This keeps you from multitasking and helps you maintain attention.

Minimize Interruptions: Reduce interruptions by disabling notifications, removing useless tabs, and setting aside specific times for focused work.

Employ the Pomodoro Technique.: Work for 25 minutes at a time in focused intervals, followed by a brief break. This method can increase output while reducing burnout.

Assign Tasks: Recognize the jobs that you can assign to others. Your time is freed up by delegation to take on tasks with a higher priority.

Batch Related Tasks: To simplify your workflow, combine related jobs. This reduces context switching and boosts productivity.

Beware of overcommitment: Regard your capabilities honestly, and try to limit the number of chores you take on. The results of overcommitting can be stress and decreased productivity.

Learn How to Say No: If a task or commitment doesn't fit with your objectives or ideals, politely decline it.

Make Good Use of Technology: Make use of apps and productivity tools to organize your projects, calendar, and reminders.

Examine and consider: Regularly evaluate your results and, if necessary, revise your strategy. Thinking back on your successes can inspire you.

Take Breaks: Plan brief rest periods during your workday. Breaks help with concentration and reduce burnout.

Establish Deadlines: Give tasks due dates to foster a sense of accountability and urgency.

Keep a healthy work-life balance: Set aside time for leisurely pursuits, downtime, and socializing. A positive work-life balance is beneficial to productivity and general well-being.

Keep in mind that productivity isn't just about getting more done; it's also about effectively allocating your time to produce worthwhile results while preserving your wellbeing. Try out several methods and tactics to see which ones suit you the best. Your success and happiness will increase as you develop vital skills in time management.

Task Prioritization: Pay Attention to What Really Matters

To effectively manage your time and accomplish your goals, prioritize your chores. Here's a step-by-step plan to help you organize your to-do list and maintain your attention on the important things.

Create a task list: Make a thorough list of all the things you have to do to get started. Include both professional and personal obligations.

Establish Relevance: Evaluate the significance of each assignment. Think about the impact each task has on your objectives, deadlines, and general wellbeing.

Bear Urgency in mind: Determine which tasks are time-sensitive or have approaching deadlines. These need to be taken care of initially.

Fourth, use the Eisenhower Matrix.

Sort tasks into the following groups:

Important and Urgent: Take care of this right away.

Plan these things for later since they are important but not urgent.

Important but Not Urgent: If you can, assign these chores to someone else.

Not Important and Not Urgent: Take into account removing or delaying these duties.

Predict Effort: Calculate the time and effort needed for each task. This enables you to set aside suitable time blocks.

Ranking by Impact: Set the chores that will have the biggest an influence on your projects, ambitions, or wellbeing as your top priorities.

Recognize Dependences: Think about tasks that require other people. Early completion of these jobs will help keep larger projects on schedule.

Simplify difficult tasks: Break down complicated activities into more manageable, smaller jobs. They become less intimidating and more manageable as a result.

Set a Maximum Number of Priorities: Choose a manageable number of the day's key priorities. Overwhelm can result from attempting to do too many chores.

Make a plan: In order to schedule time for crucial work and prevent last-minute rushes, review your forthcoming days and weeks.

Adjust as Necessary: Be adaptable and shift your priorities in response to fresh information, developments, and unanticipated occurrences.

Employ tools: Use calendars, apps, and task management tools to help you organize and prioritize your activities.

Continually Examine: Review and modify your work list and priorities from time to time. What mattered yesterday might not matter as much now.

When possible, delegate: Give others the responsibility for duties that they can handle to free up your time for more important obligations.

Take Care of Yourself: Don't forget to prioritize self-care activities. Taking care of yourself makes it easier for you to complete other responsibilities successfully.

Keep in mind that setting effective priorities requires practice. To adapt to shifting conditions and objectives, it necessitates routine examination and modifications. Making the most of your time and achieving significant outcomes may both be done by concentrating on what really counts.

Effective Breaks at Work: Boost Your Productivity

Planning your breaks wisely can really improve your workday's productivity, creativity, and general wellbeing. The following tips can help you build productive work breaks into your schedule:

Brief, Regular Breaks: Every 60 to 90 minutes, take a brief break. You may avoid burnout and keep attention by taking these quick breaks.

Move Your Body: Utilize breaks to engage in physical activity. To improve blood flow and energy levels, stretch, go for a short stroll, or do a fast workout.

Intentional Breathing: To clear your thoughts and relieve tension, try deep breathing or mindfulness activities.

Modify Your Setting: Either go outside or simply change rooms. Changing your environment might help you reenergize your mind.

Drink water and eat well: Stay hydrated and recharge your energy by drinking water and eating a nutritious snack.

Turn off the screens: Leave your computer and other screens alone. Take a rest from your eyes and mind.

Adhere to the rule of 20-20-20: Look at something 20 feet away for at least 20 seconds every 20 minutes. This lessens the effects of extended screen use on the eyes.

Socialize: Make contact with coworkers, even for a moment. A sense of community can be fostered and mood elevated through conversation.

Intentional Eating: If you're having lunch, take your time and eat slowly. Take a moment to relax and enjoy your meal.

Take a nap: If you can, get some sleep for 0–20 minutes. A brief snooze can increase focus and alertness.

Take Part in a Creative Task: Play with your favorite creative hobby for a short while. This can pique your interest and give you a mental break.

Take a Music Break: To refresh your thoughts and improve your spirits, listen to tranquil or uplifting music.

Read and write journal: Try reading a few chapters or writing down your ideas in a journal. Your attention may be drawn from work-related duties as a result of this.

Set break times: Make sure you take regular rests by setting timers. This keeps you from being overly absorbed in your work.

Relax: Take advantage of extended breaks to unwind with activities like meditation, nature walks, or brief mindfulness practices.

Keep in mind that productive breaks should provide you a mental and physical rest so you can come back to your work with renewed focus and vigor. Find what works best for you by experimenting with various hobbies, and make an effort to schedule breaks into your workday.

Getting Professional Assistance

It takes bravery and can be quite helpful to choose to get expert assistance when dealing with problems that seem overwhelming or chronic. Here is a guide on knowing when and how to ask a mental health expert for help:

Identify Signs: Consider seeking professional assistance if you consistently feel depressed, anxious, or have other emotional distress that interferes with your everyday life.

Eliminate Stigma: Keep in mind that asking for assistance indicates strength, not weakness. A mental health practitioner can help with emotional well-being in the same way that a doctor can help with physical issues.

Speak Up: Start by discussing your feelings with your health care physician or another trustworthy person. They can suggest qualified mental health specialists.

Different Professions: Psychologists, psychiatrists, counselors, and therapists are among the mental health specialists. Each has unique specialties and treatment philosophies.

Research: Look up local experts or think about internet counseling choices. Find professionals who focus on the problems you're having.

Identify Compatibility: Set up first consultations to determine whether you get along with the professional. It's important to feel at ease and understood.

Be aware of various methods: Different therapists employ different therapeutic philosophies. Some utilize psychoanalysis or mindfulness-based therapy, while others concentrate on cognitive-behavioral strategies.

Group versus individual therapy: Think about if group therapy would be more appropriate for you if you prefer individual therapy. Each choice has particular advantages.

Medicine: A psychiatrist may recommend medication as part of your treatment plan if it is appropriate. This might be suggested in addition to therapy.

Have reasonable expectations: The process of therapy demands dedication and time. Although development may not be immediate, that is not the intention.

Maintaining privacy: Confidential interactions with mental health specialists provide a safe environment for discussing your worries.

Active Involvement: Engage fully in each session of therapy. Successful outcomes depend on open communication and a desire to complete homework assignments.

Follow-Up and Upkeep: Even after you start to feel better, think about scheduling regular check-ins to preserve your wellbeing and deal with any new difficulties.

Trust Your Gut Feelings: A mental health expert may be a suitable fit for you if you have a strong relationship with them and trust them.

Be Consistent: Each person's path to better mental health is different. Be patient with the process and with yourself.

It's important to keep in mind that getting professional assistance is a powerful step toward greater mental and emotional wellbeing. Professionals are qualified to offer advice and assistance, assisting you in overcoming obstacles and creating plans for a better life.

Getting Medical Advice: Making Your Health a Priority

Consultation with a healthcare expert is essential for appropriate diagnosis, treatment, and preventive care when it comes to your physical health. Here is a guide to help you determine when and how to ask a healthcare expert for advice:

Consistent Checkups: Make regular appointments with your primary care physician for checkups. These checkups can identify any health problems early.

Address any issues: Consult a healthcare provider right away if you have any particular health issues or symptoms. They are able to offer advice and suggestions.

Be aware of your family's past: Know the medical history of your family; some diseases may run in families. Healthcare providers can use this information to evaluate your risk factors.

Specialist Suggestions: Your primary care physician might recommend you to a specialist, such as a dermatologist, cardiologist, or endocrinologist, if they discover a specific problem.

Health Education: Be sure to get the appropriate exams and shots to avoid any potential health issues.

Be frank and truthful: Give precise details about your symptoms, medical background, and way of life. This supports the decision-making of healthcare providers.

Talk about medications: To make sure your prescriptions and dietary supplements are safe and effective, talk to your doctor about them.

Ask inquiries: Do not be afraid to inquire about your health and available treatments. You get the ability to make wise selections when you are aware of your condition.

Comply with Health Advice: Follow the guidelines and recommendations that your healthcare provider has given you. This guarantees the best outcomes and well-being.

Keep Records: Observe your medical background, test outcomes, and scheduled appointments. Future consultations may find this material useful.

Get further opinions: You can gain clarity and peace of mind by getting a second opinion if you're unsure about a diagnosis or treatment plan.

Medical Assistance: Seek prompt medical help if a sudden or serious health problem arises, whether it be from your regular care physician, an urgent care center, or an emergency department.

Telemedicine: For less urgent issues, think about telemedicine options. For some diseases, virtual consultations can be practical and helpful.

Lifestyle Suggestions: On how to maintain a healthy lifestyle through nutrition, exercise, and stress reduction, healthcare professionals can offer advice.

Follow Your Gut Feelings: Whenever something about your health doesn't feel right, follow your gut and get help from a specialist.

Keep in mind that getting advice from medical specialists is a responsible and proactive move because your health is a top responsibility. Your general health and longevity can be improved by scheduling timely consultations and routine checkups.

Understanding and Treating Medical Conditions

Although diagnosing medical disorders is best left to trained healthcare professionals, being aware of probable symptoms and indicators might aid you in getting timely medical care. A guide to understanding how to spot potential medical issues is provided below:

Be Body Aware: Be aware of any changes in your bodily or emotional well-being. Important hints might be gained from your body's messages.

Inform Yourself: Discover the signs of various medical diseases. Being informed can help you see potential problems.

Family background: Be informed about any inherited medical issues. Your risk may be increased by genetic predisposition.

Track Symptoms: Keep a record of any symptoms that persist or are out of the ordinary, such as discomfort, exhaustion, hunger changes, mood swings, or weight changes.

Get Medical Help: Consult a medical expert if you have symptoms that worry you. They can offer accurate diagnosis and direction.

Avoid Self-Diagnosis: While being knowledgeable is important, refrain from self-diagnosing based simply on internet research. Accurate assessments are something that healthcare practitioners are taught to do.

Pay Attention to Your Body: Embrace your gut feeling. To rule out or solve any problems, seek medical attention if something doesn't feel right.

Continual Checkups: Make routine consultations with your primary care physician to discuss your health and receive preventive screenings.

Quick action: If you experience severe symptoms or unexpected changes in your health, don't wait to get help.

Obtain a Second Opinion: Consider getting a second opinion from a different healthcare provider if you're unsure about a diagnosis or treatment plan.

Use credible sources: Use trusted medical websites and resources while looking up symptoms online to prevent being misinformed.

Speak with experts: Consider speaking with a specialist for a more precise diagnosis if your symptoms match a particular medical condition.

Keep Lifestyle Factors in Mind: Your general health can be impacted by lifestyle decisions like nutrition, exercise, sleep, and stress management, which can also exacerbate some medical disorders.

Be Honest with Medical Personnel: Inform your healthcare professional of all pertinent details, including any changes to your routine or way of life and any worries you may have.

Take Care of Yourself: Put your health and wellbeing first by leading a healthy lifestyle. Some medical disorders can be prevented and managed with good self-care practices.

Keep in mind that diagnosing medical disorders calls for specialized knowledge from qualified individuals. While it's vital to keep informed, getting the right medical advice is essential for accurate diagnosis, effective treatment, and continuing health management.

Conclusion

Your path to improve your general well-being has been thorough thanks to "Energize Your Life: Navigating Wellness and Beating Fatigue." You have studied several methods to deal with exhaustion, enhance mental and emotional well-being, control stress, and place a high priority on self-care throughout these chapters. You now understand how critical it is to ask for help, build meaningful relationships, and organize your time and activities well.

Keep in mind that achieving well-being requires constant effort. It represents a dedication to protecting your physical, mental, and emotional wellbeing. You have the means to build a more well-balanced, energised, and fulfilling life by putting the insights and strategies discussed in this manual into practice.

Continue to put self-care first as you go forward, adopt new habits, and look for the help you require. Your route to well-being is entirely personal, whether it involves developing healthier behaviors, practicing mindfulness, getting help from a professional, or just carving out time for enjoyable activities.

We are grateful that you chose to travel this path with "Energize Your Life: Navigating Wellness and Beating

Fatigue." As you put your health first in all aspect of your life, may you flourish, find energy, and rediscover your sense of purpose.

An Integrative Guide to Wellness Navigation

The comprehensive manual "Energize Your Life: Navigating Wellness and Beating Fatigue" was created to give you the information and resources you need to improve your general well-being. You have studied a wide range of subjects in the chapters, from preventing weariness and comprehending its origins to fostering mental and emotional well-being, controlling stress, and efficiently managing your time and tasks.

You now understand the importance of getting help, making relationships, and taking care of yourself. This guide has offered practical advice for every element of your well-being, from prioritizing sleep, nutrition, and exercise to learning mindfulness techniques and getting help from a professional when necessary.

Keep in mind that achieving and maintaining well-being calls for effort, consciousness, and dedication. You can enjoy more energy, less stress, more mental clarity, and an overall higher standard of living by adopting the advice from this book into your daily life.

"Energize Your Life: Navigating Wellness and Beating Fatigue" is a helpful tool that gives you the power to take control of your well-being, whether you're looking for strategies to reduce fatigue, manage stress, practice mindfulness, or develop a balanced lifestyle. Take up these habits and set out on a path to a healthier, happier, and more contented you.